*This Journal belongs to:*

_____

There is a saying - you can't manage what you don't measure.

Measuring your intake helps you manage your output.

A healthier inside makes for a more attractive outside.

Become your own Boss
today, by managing
what you eat, and how
you use those calories

# Tips for using a habit tracker

- **Why**

    - Here a five compelling reasons.
    - 1. It creates a visual cue that can remind you to act.
    - 2. It is motivating to see the progress you are making.
    - 3. It motivates you to continue.
    - 4. It provides immediate satisfaction.
    - 5. Finally, tracking feels rewarding
- Tracking specific habits also helps keep you focused on the process rather
- than the result.

- **What**
-
- **Common habits to track:**
- meditate
- write 1 thing I'm grateful for
- Exercise
- Walk the dog

- **When**
- Anytime you remember really but it has been found for some that )
-

# Habit Tracker

Month _____

Year

| Day | Write in Journal | Meditate | Exercise | | | | | | | | | | | |
|-----|------|------|------|---|---|---|---|---|---|---|---|---|---|---|
| 1 | ▓ | | ▓ | | | | | | | | | | | |
| 2 | | ▓ | | | | | | | | | | | | |
| 3 | ▓ | ▓ | | | | | | | | | | | | |
| 4 | | ▓ | | | | | | | | | | | | |
| 5 | ▓ | | ▓ | | | | | | | | | | | |
| 6 | | ▓ | ▓ | | | | | | | | | | | |
| 7 | ▓ | | | | | | | | | | | | | |
| 8 | | | | | | | | | | | | | | |
| 9 | | | | | | | | | | | | | | |
| 10 | | | | | | | | | | | | | | |
| 11 | | | | | | | | | | | | | | |
| 12 | | | | | | | | | | | | | | |
| 13 | | | | | | | | | | | | | | |
| 14 | | | | | | | | | | | | | | |
| 15 | | | | | | | | | | | | | | |
| 16 | | | | | | | | | | | | | | |
| 17 | | | | | | | | | | | | | | |
| 18 | | | | | | | | | | | | | | |
| 19 | | | | | | | | | | | | | | |
| 20 | | | | | | | | | | | | | | |
| 21 | | | | | | | | | | | | | | |
| 22 | | | | | | | | | | | | | | |
| 23 | | | | | | | | | | | | | | |
| 24 | | | | | | | | | | | | | | |
| 25 | | | | | | | | | | | | | | |
| 26 | | | | | | | | | | | | | | |
| 27 | | | | | | | | | | | | | | |
| 28 | | | | | | | | | | | | | | |
| 29 | | | | | | | | | | | | | | |
| 30 | | | | | | | | | | | | | | |
| 31 | | | | | | | | | | | | | | |

# Habit
# Tracker

Month _____

Year

| ay | | | | | | | | | | | | | | |
|----|--|--|--|--|--|--|--|--|--|--|--|--|--|--|
| 2 | | | | | | | | | | | | | | |
| 3 | | | | | | | | | | | | | | |
| 4 | | | | | | | | | | | | | | |
| 5 | | | | | | | | | | | | | | |
| 6 | | | | | | | | | | | | | | |
| 7 | | | | | | | | | | | | | | |
| 8 | | | | | | | | | | | | | | |
| 9 | | | | | | | | | | | | | | |
| 0 | | | | | | | | | | | | | | |
| 1 | | | | | | | | | | | | | | |
| 2 | | | | | | | | | | | | | | |
| 3 | | | | | | | | | | | | | | |
| 4 | | | | | | | | | | | | | | |
| 5 | | | | | | | | | | | | | | |
| 6 | | | | | | | | | | | | | | |
| 7 | | | | | | | | | | | | | | |
| 8 | | | | | | | | | | | | | | |
| 9 | | | | | | | | | | | | | | |
| 20 | | | | | | | | | | | | | | |
| 1 | | | | | | | | | | | | | | |
| 22 | | | | | | | | | | | | | | |
| 23 | | | | | | | | | | | | | | |
| 24 | | | | | | | | | | | | | | |
| 25 | | | | | | | | | | | | | | |
| 26 | | | | | | | | | | | | | | |
| 27 | | | | | | | | | | | | | | |
| 28 | | | | | | | | | | | | | | |
| 29 | | | | | | | | | | | | | | |
| 30 | | | | | | | | | | | | | | |
| 31 | | | | | | | | | | | | | | |

Notes:

| Date | | S  M  T  W  T  F  S | |
|---|---|---|---|
| **Breakfast** | | Amount | Calories (kcal) |
| | | | |
| | | | |
| | | | |
| | | | |
| | | Total | |
| **Snack** | | Amount | Calories (kcal) |
| | | | |
| | | | |
| | | | |
| | | | |
| | | | |
| | | Total | |
| **Lunch** | | Amount | Calories (kcal) |
| | | | |
| | | | |
| | | | |
| | | | |
| | | | |
| | | Total | |

| Snack | Amount | Calories (kcal) |
|---|---|---|
| | | |
| | | |
| | | |
| | Total | |
| **Dinner** | Amount | Calories (kcal) |
| | | |
| | | |
| | | |
| | | |
| | | |
| | | |
| | | |
| | Total | |
| **Snack** | Amount | Calories (kcal) |
| | | |
| | | |
| | | |
| | Total | |
| **Exercise** | Duration | Calories burned (kcal) |
| | | |
| | | |
| | | |
| **Water** | | | | | | | | | Fruit & Veggies | | | | | | | | |

Notes:

| Date | S M T W T F S | |
|---|---|---|
| **Breakfast** | Amount | Calories (kcal) |
| | | |
| | | |
| | | |
| | | |
| | | |
| | Total | |
| **Snack** | Amount | Calories (kcal) |
| | | |
| | | |
| | | |
| | | |
| | | |
| | | |
| | Total | |
| **Lunch** | Amount | Calories (kcal) |
| | | |
| | | |
| | | |
| | | |
| | | |
| | | |
| | Total | |

| Snack | Amount | Calories (kcal) |
|---|---|---|
| | | |
| | | |
| | | |
| | Total | |
| **Dinner** | Amount | Calories (kcal) |
| | | |
| | | |
| | | |
| | | |
| | | |
| | | |
| | Total | |
| **Snack** | Amount | Calories (kcal) |
| | | |
| | | |
| | | |
| | Total | |
| **Exercise** | Duration | Calories burned (kcal) |
| | | |
| | | |
| | | |
| **Water** | Fruit & Veggies | |

Notes:

| Date | | S M T W T F S | |
|---|---|---|---|
| **Breakfast** | Amount | Calories (kcal) | |
| | | | |
| | | | |
| | | | |
| | | | |
| | | | |
| | Total | | |
| **Snack** | Amount | Calories (kcal) | |
| | | | |
| | | | |
| | | | |
| | | | |
| | | | |
| | | | |
| | Total | | |
| **Lunch** | Amount | Calories (kcal) | |
| | | | |
| | | | |
| | | | |
| | | | |
| | | | |
| | Total | | |

| Snack | Amount | Calories (kcal) |
|---|---|---|
| | | |
| | | |
| | | |
| | Total | |
| **Dinner** | Amount | Calories (kcal) |
| | | |
| | | |
| | | |
| | | |
| | | |
| | | |
| | | |
| | Total | |
| **Snack** | Amount | Calories (kcal) |
| | | |
| | | |
| | | |
| | Total | |
| **Exercise** | Duration | Calories burned (kcal) |
| | | |
| | | |
| | | |
| **Water** | | | | | | | | | Fruit & Veggies | | | | | | | | |

Notes:

| Date | | S  M  T  W  T  F  S | |
|---|---|---|---|
| **Breakfast** | | Amount | Calories (kcal) |
| | | | |
| | | | |
| | | | |
| | | | |
| | | Total | |
| **Snack** | | Amount | Calories (kcal) |
| | | | |
| | | | |
| | | | |
| | | | |
| | | | |
| | | Total | |
| **Lunch** | | Amount | Calories (kcal) |
| | | | |
| | | | |
| | | | |
| | | | |
| | | | |
| | | Total | |

| Snack | Amount | Calories (kcal) |
|---|---|---|
| | | |
| | | |
| | | |
| | Total | |
| Dinner | Amount | Calories (kcal) |
| | | |
| | | |
| | | |
| | | |
| | | |
| | | |
| | | |
| | Total | |
| Snack | Amount | Calories (kcal) |
| | | |
| | | |
| | | |
| | Total | |
| Exercise | Duration | Calories burned (kcal) |
| | | |
| | | |
| | | |

| Water | | | | | | | | Fruit & Veggies | | | | | | | |
|---|---|---|---|---|---|---|---|---|---|---|---|---|---|---|---|

Notes:

| Date | | S  M  T  W  T  F  S |
|---|---|---|
| **Breakfast** | Amount | Calories (kcal) |
| | | |
| | | |
| | | |
| | | |
| | Total | |
| **Snack** | Amount | Calories (kcal) |
| | | |
| | | |
| | | |
| | | |
| | | |
| | | |
| | Total | |
| **Lunch** | Amount | Calories (kcal) |
| | | |
| | | |
| | | |
| | | |
| | | |
| | | |
| | Total | |

| Snack | Amount | Calories (kcal) |
|---|---|---|
|  |  |  |
|  |  |  |
|  |  |  |
|  | Total |  |
| **Dinner** | Amount | Calories (kcal) |
|  |  |  |
|  |  |  |
|  |  |  |
|  |  |  |
|  |  |  |
|  |  |  |
|  | Total |  |
| **Snack** | Amount | Calories (kcal) |
|  |  |  |
|  |  |  |
|  |  |  |
|  | Total |  |
| **Exercise** | Duration | Calories burned (kcal) |
|  |  |  |
|  |  |  |
|  |  |  |
| **Water** |  | Fruit & Veggies |  |

Notes:

| Date | | S  M  T  W  T  F  S | |
|---|---|---|---|
| **Breakfast** | | Amount | Calories (kcal) |
| | | | |
| | | | |
| | | | |
| | | | |
| | | Total | |
| **Snack** | | Amount | Calories (kcal) |
| | | | |
| | | | |
| | | | |
| | | | |
| | | | |
| | | | |
| | | Total | |
| **Lunch** | | Amount | Calories (kcal) |
| | | | |
| | | | |
| | | | |
| | | | |
| | | | |
| | | | |
| | | Total | |

| Snack | Amount | Calories (kcal) |
|---|---|---|
| | | |
| | | |
| | | |
| | Total | |
| **Dinner** | Amount | Calories (kcal) |
| | | |
| | | |
| | | |
| | | |
| | | |
| | | |
| | | |
| | Total | |
| **Snack** | Amount | Calories (kcal) |
| | | |
| | | |
| | | |
| | Total | |
| **Exercise** | Duration | Calories burned (kcal) |
| | | |
| | | |
| | | |
| **Water** | | | | | | | | Fruit & Veggies | | | | | | | |

Notes:

| Date | | S  M  T  W  T  F  S | |
|---|---|---|---|
| **Breakfast** | | Amount | Calories (kcal) |
| | | | |
| | | | |
| | | | |
| | | | |
| | | | |
| | | Total | |
| **Snack** | | Amount | Calories (kcal) |
| | | | |
| | | | |
| | | | |
| | | | |
| | | | |
| | | Total | |
| **Lunch** | | Amount | Calories (kcal) |
| | | | |
| | | | |
| | | | |
| | | | |
| | | | |
| | | Total | |

| Snack | Amount | Calories (kcal) |
|---|---|---|
|  |  |  |
|  |  |  |
|  |  |  |
|  | Total |  |
| Dinner | Amount | Calories (kcal) |
|  |  |  |
|  |  |  |
|  |  |  |
|  |  |  |
|  |  |  |
|  |  |  |
|  | Total |  |
| Snack | Amount | Calories (kcal) |
|  |  |  |
|  |  |  |
|  |  |  |
|  | Total |  |
| Exercise | Duration | Calories burned (kcal) |
|  |  |  |
|  |  |  |
|  |  |  |

| Water | | | | | | | | Fruit & Veggies | | | | | | | | |

Notes:

| Date | S M T W T F S | |
|---|---|---|
| **Breakfast** | Amount | Calories (kcal) |
| | | |
| | | |
| | | |
| | | |
| | | |
| | Total | |
| **Snack** | Amount | Calories (kcal) |
| | | |
| | | |
| | | |
| | | |
| | | |
| | | |
| | Total | |
| **Lunch** | Amount | Calories (kcal) |
| | | |
| | | |
| | | |
| | | |
| | | |
| | | |
| | Total | |

| Snack | Amount | Calories (kcal) |
|---|---|---|
| | | |
| | | |
| | | |
| | Total | |
| **Dinner** | Amount | Calories (kcal) |
| | | |
| | | |
| | | |
| | | |
| | | |
| | | |
| | Total | |
| **Snack** | Amount | Calories (kcal) |
| | | |
| | | |
| | Total | |
| **Exercise** | Duration | Calories burned (kcal) |
| | | |
| | | |
| | | |
| **Water** | Fruit & Veggies | |

# Notes:

| Date | S M T W T F S | |
|---|---|---|
| **Breakfast** | Amount | Calories (kcal) |
| | | |
| | | |
| | | |
| | | |
| | Total | |
| **Snack** | Amount | Calories (kcal) |
| | | |
| | | |
| | | |
| | | |
| | | |
| | Total | |
| **Lunch** | Amount | Calories (kcal) |
| | | |
| | | |
| | | |
| | | |
| | | |
| | Total | |

| Snack | Amount | Calories (kcal) |
|---|---|---|
|  |  |  |
|  |  |  |
|  |  |  |
|  | Total |  |
| **Dinner** | Amount | Calories (kcal) |
|  |  |  |
|  |  |  |
|  |  |  |
|  |  |  |
|  |  |  |
|  |  |  |
|  |  |  |
|  | Total |  |
| **Snack** | Amount | Calories (kcal) |
|  |  |  |
|  |  |  |
|  |  |  |
|  | Total |  |
| **Exercise** | Duration | Calories burned (kcal) |
|  |  |  |
|  |  |  |
|  |  |  |
| **Water** | | | | | | | | Fruit & Veggies | | | | | | | |

Notes:

| Date | | S  M  T  W  T  F  S | |
|---|---|---|---|
| **Breakfast** | | Amount | Calories (kcal) |
| | | | |
| | | | |
| | | | |
| | | | |
| | | Total | |
| **Snack** | | Amount | Calories (kcal) |
| | | | |
| | | | |
| | | | |
| | | | |
| | | | |
| | | Total | |
| **Lunch** | | Amount | Calories (kcal) |
| | | | |
| | | | |
| | | | |
| | | | |
| | | | |
| | | Total | |

| Snack | Amount | Calories (kcal) |
|---|---|---|
|  |  |  |
|  |  |  |
|  |  |  |
|  | Total |  |
| **Dinner** | Amount | Calories (kcal) |
|  |  |  |
|  |  |  |
|  |  |  |
|  |  |  |
|  |  |  |
|  |  |  |
|  | Total |  |
| **Snack** | Amount | Calories (kcal) |
|  |  |  |
|  |  |  |
|  | Total |  |
| **Exercise** | Duration | Calories burned (kcal) |
|  |  |  |
|  |  |  |
|  |  |  |
| **Water** | Fruit & Veggies |  |

Notes:

| Date | S M T W T F S | |
|---|---|---|
| **Breakfast** | Amount | Calories (kcal) |
| | | |
| | | |
| | | |
| | | |
| | | |
| | Total | |
| **Snack** | Amount | Calories (kcal) |
| | | |
| | | |
| | | |
| | | |
| | | |
| | Total | |
| **Lunch** | Amount | Calories (kcal) |
| | | |
| | | |
| | | |
| | | |
| | | |
| | Total | |

| Snack | Amount | Calories (kcal) |
|---|---|---|
| | | |
| | | |
| | | |
| | Total | |
| **Dinner** | Amount | Calories (kcal) |
| | | |
| | | |
| | | |
| | | |
| | | |
| | | |
| | Total | |
| **Snack** | Amount | Calories (kcal) |
| | | |
| | | |
| | | |
| | Total | |
| **Exercise** | Duration | Calories burned (kcal) |
| | | |
| | | |
| | | |
| **Water** | | | | | | | | Fruit & Veggies | | | | | | | |

Notes:

| Date | | S  M  T  W  T  F  S | |
|---|---|---|---|
| **Breakfast** | Amount | | Calories (kcal) |
| | | | |
| | | | |
| | | | |
| | | | |
| | Total | | |
| **Snack** | Amount | | Calories (kcal) |
| | | | |
| | | | |
| | | | |
| | | | |
| | | | |
| | Total | | |
| **Lunch** | Amount | | Calories (kcal) |
| | | | |
| | | | |
| | | | |
| | | | |
| | | | |
| | Total | | |

| Snack | Amount | Calories (kcal) |
| --- | --- | --- |
| | | |
| | | |
| | | |
| | Total | |
| Dinner | Amount | Calories (kcal) |
| | | |
| | | |
| | | |
| | | |
| | | |
| | | |
| | Total | |
| Snack | Amount | Calories (kcal) |
| | | |
| | | |
| | | |
| | Total | |
| Exercise | Duration | Calories burned (kcal) |
| | | |
| | | |
| | | |

| Water | | | | | | | | Fruit & Veggies | | | | | | | |
| --- | --- | --- | --- | --- | --- | --- | --- | --- | --- | --- | --- | --- | --- | --- | --- |

Notes:

| Date | S M T W T F S | |
|---|---|---|
| **Breakfast** | Amount | Calories (kcal) |
| | | |
| | | |
| | | |
| | | |
| | Total | |
| **Snack** | Amount | Calories (kcal) |
| | | |
| | | |
| | | |
| | | |
| | | |
| | Total | |
| **Lunch** | Amount | Calories (kcal) |
| | | |
| | | |
| | | |
| | | |
| | | |
| | Total | |

| Snack | Amount | Calories (kcal) |
|---|---|---|
| | | |
| | | |
| | | |
| | Total | |
| Dinner | Amount | Calories (kcal) |
| | | |
| | | |
| | | |
| | | |
| | | |
| | | |
| | Total | |
| Snack | Amount | Calories (kcal) |
| | | |
| | | |
| | | |
| | Total | |
| Exercise | Duration | Calories burned (kcal) |
| | | |
| | | |
| | | |
| Water | | Fruit & Veggies | |

Notes:

| Date | | S M T W T F S |
|---|---|---|
| **Breakfast** | Amount | Calories (kcal) |
| | | |
| | | |
| | | |
| | | |
| | Total | |
| **Snack** | Amount | Calories (kcal) |
| | | |
| | | |
| | | |
| | | |
| | | |
| | Total | |
| **Lunch** | Amount | Calories (kcal) |
| | | |
| | | |
| | | |
| | | |
| | | |
| | Total | |

| Snack | Amount | Calories (kcal) |
|---|---|---|
| | | |
| | | |
| | | |
| | Total | |
| **Dinner** | Amount | Calories (kcal) |
| | | |
| | | |
| | | |
| | | |
| | | |
| | | |
| | | |
| | Total | |
| **Snack** | Amount | Calories (kcal) |
| | | |
| | | |
| | | |
| | Total | |
| **Exercise** | Duration | Calories burned (kcal) |
| | | |
| | | |
| | | |
| **Water** | | | | | | | | | Fruit & Veggies | | | | | | | | |

Notes:

| Date | S M T W T F S | |
|---|---|---|
| **Breakfast** | Amount | Calories (kcal) |
| | | |
| | | |
| | | |
| | | |
| | | |
| | Total | |
| **Snack** | Amount | Calories (kcal) |
| | | |
| | | |
| | | |
| | | |
| | | |
| | Total | |
| **Lunch** | Amount | Calories (kcal) |
| | | |
| | | |
| | | |
| | | |
| | | |
| | Total | |

| Snack | Amount | Calories (kcal) |
|---|---|---|
| | | |
| | | |
| | | |
| | Total | |
| **Dinner** | Amount | Calories (kcal) |
| | | |
| | | |
| | | |
| | | |
| | | |
| | | |
| | | |
| | Total | |
| **Snack** | Amount | Calories (kcal) |
| | | |
| | | |
| | | |
| | Total | |
| **Exercise** | Duration | Calories burned (kcal) |
| | | |
| | | |
| | | |
| **Water** | Fruit & Veggies | |

Notes:

| Date | | S  M  T  W  T  F  S |
|---|---|---|
| **Breakfast** | Amount | Calories (kcal) |
| | | |
| | | |
| | | |
| | | |
| | Total | |
| **Snack** | Amount | Calories (kcal) |
| | | |
| | | |
| | | |
| | | |
| | | |
| | | |
| | Total | |
| **Lunch** | Amount | Calories (kcal) |
| | | |
| | | |
| | | |
| | | |
| | | |
| | Total | |

| Snack | Amount | Calories (kcal) |
|---|---|---|
| | | |
| | | |
| | Total | |
| Dinner | Amount | Calories (kcal) |
| | | |
| | | |
| | | |
| | | |
| | | |
| | | |
| | Total | |
| Snack | Amount | Calories (kcal) |
| | | |
| | | |
| | Total | |
| Exercise | Duration | Calories burned (kcal) |
| | | |
| | | |
| | | |

| Water | | | | | | | | | Fruit & Veggies | | | | | | | |
|---|---|---|---|---|---|---|---|---|---|---|---|---|---|---|---|---|

Notes:

| Date | | S M T W T F S | |
|---|---|---|---|
| **Breakfast** | Amount | Calories (kcal) | |
| | | | |
| | | | |
| | | | |
| | | | |
| | | | |
| | Total | | |
| **Snack** | Amount | Calories (kcal) | |
| | | | |
| | | | |
| | | | |
| | | | |
| | | | |
| | | | |
| | Total | | |
| **Lunch** | Amount | Calories (kcal) | |
| | | | |
| | | | |
| | | | |
| | | | |
| | | | |
| | | | |
| | Total | | |

| Snack | Amount | Calories (kcal) |
|---|---|---|
| | | |
| | | |
| | | |
| | Total | |
| Dinner | Amount | Calories (kcal) |
| | | |
| | | |
| | | |
| | | |
| | | |
| | | |
| | Total | |
| Snack | Amount | Calories (kcal) |
| | | |
| | | |
| | Total | |
| Exercise | Duration | Calories burned (kcal) |
| | | |
| | | |
| | | |
| Water | | | | | | | | Fruit & Veggies | | | | | | | |

Notes:

| Date | | S M T W T F S |
|---|---|---|
| **Breakfast** | Amount | Calories (kcal) |
| | | |
| | | |
| | | |
| | | |
| | | |
| | Total | |
| **Snack** | Amount | Calories (kcal) |
| | | |
| | | |
| | | |
| | | |
| | | |
| | | |
| | Total | |
| **Lunch** | Amount | Calories (kcal) |
| | | |
| | | |
| | | |
| | | |
| | | |
| | | |
| | Total | |

| Snack | Amount | Calories (kcal) |
|---|---|---|
| | | |
| | | |
| | | |
| | Total | |
| **Dinner** | Amount | Calories (kcal) |
| | | |
| | | |
| | | |
| | | |
| | | |
| | | |
| | Total | |
| **Snack** | Amount | Calories (kcal) |
| | | |
| | | |
| | | |
| | Total | |
| **Exercise** | Duration | Calories burned (kcal) |
| | | |
| | | |
| | | |
| **Water** | Fruit & Veggies | |

Notes:

| Date | | S M T W T F S | |
|---|---|---|---|
| **Breakfast** | Amount | Calories (kcal) | |
| | | | |
| | | | |
| | | | |
| | | | |
| | | | |
| | Total | | |
| **Snack** | Amount | Calories (kcal) | |
| | | | |
| | | | |
| | | | |
| | | | |
| | | | |
| | | | |
| | Total | | |
| **Lunch** | Amount | Calories (kcal) | |
| | | | |
| | | | |
| | | | |
| | | | |
| | | | |
| | Total | | |

| Snack | Amount | Calories (kcal) |
|---|---|---|
| | | |
| | | |
| | | |
| | Total | |
| **Dinner** | Amount | Calories (kcal) |
| | | |
| | | |
| | | |
| | | |
| | | |
| | | |
| | Total | |
| **Snack** | Amount | Calories (kcal) |
| | | |
| | | |
| | | |
| | Total | |
| **Exercise** | Duration | Calories burned (kcal) |
| | | |
| | | |
| | | |
| **Water** | Fruit & Veggies | |

Notes:

| Date | | S  M  T  W  T  F  S |
|---|---|---|
| **Breakfast** | Amount | Calories (kcal) |
| | | |
| | | |
| | | |
| | | |
| | | |
| | Total | |
| **Snack** | Amount | Calories (kcal) |
| | | |
| | | |
| | | |
| | | |
| | | |
| | | |
| | Total | |
| **Lunch** | Amount | Calories (kcal) |
| | | |
| | | |
| | | |
| | | |
| | | |
| | | |
| | Total | |

| Snack | Amount | Calories (kcal) |
|---|---|---|
| | | |
| | | |
| | | |
| | Total | |
| **Dinner** | Amount | Calories (kcal) |
| | | |
| | | |
| | | |
| | | |
| | | |
| | | |
| | Total | |
| **Snack** | Amount | Calories (kcal) |
| | | |
| | | |
| | | |
| | Total | |
| **Exercise** | Duration | Calories burned (kcal) |
| | | |
| | | |
| | | |
| **Water** | Fruit & Veggies | |

Notes:

| Date | | S  M  T  W  T  F  S | |
|---|---|---|---|
| **Breakfast** | Amount | | Calories (kcal) |
| | | | |
| | | | |
| | | | |
| | | | |
| | Total | | |
| **Snack** | Amount | | Calories (kcal) |
| | | | |
| | | | |
| | | | |
| | | | |
| | | | |
| | | | |
| | Total | | |
| **Lunch** | Amount | | Calories (kcal) |
| | | | |
| | | | |
| | | | |
| | | | |
| | | | |
| | Total | | |

| Snack | Amount | Calories (kcal) |
|---|---|---|
| | | |
| | | |
| | | |
| | Total | |
| **Dinner** | Amount | Calories (kcal) |
| | | |
| | | |
| | | |
| | | |
| | | |
| | | |
| | | |
| | Total | |
| **Snack** | Amount | Calories (kcal) |
| | | |
| | | |
| | | |
| | Total | |
| **Exercise** | Duration | Calories burned (kcal) |
| | | |
| | | |
| | | |
| **Water** | Fruit & Veggies | |

Notes:

| Date | | S M T W T F S | |
|---|---|---|---|
| **Breakfast** | Amount | | Calories (kcal) |
| | | | |
| | | | |
| | | | |
| | | | |
| | Total | | |
| **Snack** | Amount | | Calories (kcal) |
| | | | |
| | | | |
| | | | |
| | | | |
| | | | |
| | | | |
| | Total | | |
| **Lunch** | Amount | | Calories (kcal) |
| | | | |
| | | | |
| | | | |
| | | | |
| | | | |
| | | | |
| | Total | | |

| Snack | Amount | Calories (kcal) |
|---|---|---|
|  |  |  |
|  |  |  |
|  | Total |  |
| **Dinner** | Amount | Calories (kcal) |
|  |  |  |
|  |  |  |
|  |  |  |
|  |  |  |
|  |  |  |
|  | Total |  |
| **Snack** | Amount | Calories (kcal) |
|  |  |  |
|  |  |  |
|  | Total |  |
| **Exercise** | Duration | Calories burned (kcal) |
|  |  |  |
|  |  |  |
| **Water** |  | Fruit & Veggies |

Notes:

| Date | | S M T W T F S | |
|---|---|---|---|
| **Breakfast** | Amount | Calories (kcal) |
| | | |
| | | |
| | | |
| | | |
| | Total | |
| **Snack** | Amount | Calories (kcal) |
| | | |
| | | |
| | | |
| | | |
| | | |
| | Total | |
| **Lunch** | Amount | Calories (kcal) |
| | | |
| | | |
| | | |
| | | |
| | | |
| | Total | |

| Snack | Amount | Calories (kcal) |
|---|---|---|
| | | |
| | | |
| | | |
| | Total | |
| Dinner | Amount | Calories (kcal) |
| | | |
| | | |
| | | |
| | | |
| | | |
| | | |
| | | |
| | Total | |
| Snack | Amount | Calories (kcal) |
| | | |
| | | |
| | | |
| | Total | |
| Exercise | Duration | Calories burned (kcal) |
| | | |
| | | |
| | | |

| Water | | | | | | | | Fruit & Veggies | | | | | | | | |
|---|---|---|---|---|---|---|---|---|---|---|---|---|---|---|---|---|

Notes:

| Date | S M T W T F S | |
|---|---|---|
| **Breakfast** | Amount | Calories (kcal) |
| | | |
| | | |
| | | |
| | | |
| | | |
| | Total | |
| **Snack** | Amount | Calories (kcal) |
| | | |
| | | |
| | | |
| | | |
| | | |
| | | |
| | Total | |
| **Lunch** | Amount | Calories (kcal) |
| | | |
| | | |
| | | |
| | | |
| | | |
| | Total | |

| Snack | Amount | Calories (kcal) |
|---|---|---|
|  |  |  |
|  |  |  |
|  |  |  |
|  | Total |  |
| **Dinner** | Amount | Calories (kcal) |
|  |  |  |
|  |  |  |
|  |  |  |
|  |  |  |
|  |  |  |
|  |  |  |
|  |  |  |
|  | Total |  |
| **Snack** | Amount | Calories (kcal) |
|  |  |  |
|  |  |  |
|  |  |  |
|  | Total |  |
| **Exercise** | Duration | Calories burned (kcal) |
|  |  |  |
|  |  |  |
|  |  |  |
| **Water** |  | Fruit & Veggies |  |

Notes:

| Date | S M T W T F S | |
|---|---|---|
| **Breakfast** | Amount | Calories (kcal) |
| | | |
| | | |
| | | |
| | | |
| | Total | |
| **Snack** | Amount | Calories (kcal) |
| | | |
| | | |
| | | |
| | | |
| | | |
| | Total | |
| **Lunch** | Amount | Calories (kcal) |
| | | |
| | | |
| | | |
| | | |
| | | |
| | Total | |

| Snack | Amount | Calories (kcal) |
|---|---|---|
|  |  |  |
|  |  |  |
|  |  |  |
|  | Total |  |
| Dinner | Amount | Calories (kcal) |
|  |  |  |
|  |  |  |
|  |  |  |
|  |  |  |
|  |  |  |
|  |  |  |
|  |  |  |
|  | Total |  |
| Snack | Amount | Calories (kcal) |
|  |  |  |
|  |  |  |
|  |  |  |
|  | Total |  |
| Exercise | Duration | Calories burned (kcal) |
|  |  |  |
|  |  |  |
|  |  |  |
| Water | | | | | | | | Fruit & Veggies | | | | | | | | |

Notes:

| Date | | S M T W T F S | |
|---|---|---|---|
| **Breakfast** | | Amount | Calories (kcal) |
| | | | |
| | | | |
| | | | |
| | | | |
| | | Total | |
| **Snack** | | Amount | Calories (kcal) |
| | | | |
| | | | |
| | | | |
| | | | |
| | | | |
| | | Total | |
| **Lunch** | | Amount | Calories (kcal) |
| | | | |
| | | | |
| | | | |
| | | | |
| | | | |
| | | Total | |

| Snack | Amount | Calories (kcal) |
|---|---|---|
| | | |
| | | |
| | | |
| | Total | |
| Dinner | Amount | Calories (kcal) |
| | | |
| | | |
| | | |
| | | |
| | | |
| | | |
| | | |
| | Total | |
| Snack | Amount | Calories (kcal) |
| | | |
| | | |
| | | |
| | Total | |
| Exercise | Duration | Calories burned (kcal) |
| | | |
| | | |
| | | |
| Water | | Fruit & Veggies | |

Notes:

| Date | | S M T W T F S | |
|---|---|---|---|
| **Breakfast** | Amount | Calories (kcal) | |
| | | | |
| | | | |
| | | | |
| | | | |
| | Total | | |
| **Snack** | Amount | Calories (kcal) | |
| | | | |
| | | | |
| | | | |
| | | | |
| | | | |
| | Total | | |
| **Lunch** | Amount | Calories (kcal) | |
| | | | |
| | | | |
| | | | |
| | | | |
| | | | |
| | Total | | |

| Snack | Amount | Calories (kcal) |
|---|---|---|
| | | |
| | | |
| | | |
| | Total | |
| Dinner | Amount | Calories (kcal) |
| | | |
| | | |
| | | |
| | | |
| | | |
| | | |
| | | |
| | Total | |
| Snack | Amount | Calories (kcal) |
| | | |
| | | |
| | | |
| | Total | |
| Exercise | Duration | Calories burned (kcal) |
| | | |
| | | |
| | | |

| Water | | | | | | | | Fruit & Veggies | | | | | | | | |
|---|---|---|---|---|---|---|---|---|---|---|---|---|---|---|---|---|

Notes:

| Date | S M T W T F S | |
|---|---|---|
| **Breakfast** | Amount | Calories (kcal) |
| | | |
| | | |
| | | |
| | | |
| | Total | |
| **Snack** | Amount | Calories (kcal) |
| | | |
| | | |
| | | |
| | | |
| | | |
| | Total | |
| **Lunch** | Amount | Calories (kcal) |
| | | |
| | | |
| | | |
| | | |
| | | |
| | Total | |

| Snack | Amount | Calories (kcal) |
|---|---|---|
| | | |
| | | |
| | | |
| | Total | |
| **Dinner** | Amount | Calories (kcal) |
| | | |
| | | |
| | | |
| | | |
| | | |
| | | |
| | Total | |
| Snack | Amount | Calories (kcal) |
| | | |
| | | |
| | Total | |
| **Exercise** | Duration | Calories burned (kcal) |
| | | |
| | | |
| | | |

| Water | | | | | | | Fruit & Veggies | | | | | | |
|---|---|---|---|---|---|---|---|---|---|---|---|---|---|

Notes:

| Date | S M T W T F S | |
|---|---|---|
| **Breakfast** | Amount | Calories (kcal) |
| | | |
| | | |
| | | |
| | | |
| | | |
| | Total | |
| **Snack** | Amount | Calories (kcal) |
| | | |
| | | |
| | | |
| | | |
| | | |
| | | |
| | Total | |
| **Lunch** | Amount | Calories (kcal) |
| | | |
| | | |
| | | |
| | | |
| | | |
| | Total | |

| Snack | Amount | Calories (kcal) |
|---|---|---|
| | | |
| | | |
| | | |
| | Total | |
| **Dinner** | Amount | Calories (kcal) |
| | | |
| | | |
| | | |
| | | |
| | | |
| | | |
| | | |
| | Total | |
| **Snack** | Amount | Calories (kcal) |
| | | |
| | | |
| | | |
| | Total | |
| **Exercise** | Duration | Calories burned (kcal) |
| | | |
| | | |
| | | |
| **Water** | Fruit & Veggies | |

Notes:

| Date | | S M T W T F S | |
|---|---|---|---|
| **Breakfast** | Amount | Calories (kcal) | |
| | | | |
| | | | |
| | | | |
| | | | |
| | | | |
| | Total | | |
| **Snack** | Amount | Calories (kcal) | |
| | | | |
| | | | |
| | | | |
| | | | |
| | | | |
| | | | |
| | Total | | |
| **Lunch** | Amount | Calories (kcal) | |
| | | | |
| | | | |
| | | | |
| | | | |
| | | | |
| | | | |
| | Total | | |

| Snack | Amount | Calories (kcal) |
|---|---|---|
| | | |
| | | |
| | | |
| | Total | |
| **Dinner** | Amount | Calories (kcal) |
| | | |
| | | |
| | | |
| | | |
| | | |
| | | |
| | Total | |
| **Snack** | Amount | Calories (kcal) |
| | | |
| | | |
| | | |
| | Total | |
| **Exercise** | Duration | Calories burned (kcal) |
| | | |
| | | |
| | | |

| Water | | | | | | | | | Fruit & Veggies | | | | | | | |
|---|---|---|---|---|---|---|---|---|---|---|---|---|---|---|---|---|

Notes:

| Date | | S M T W T F S | |
|---|---|---|---|
| **Breakfast** | Amount | Calories (kcal) | |
| | | | |
| | | | |
| | | | |
| | | | |
| | Total | | |
| **Snack** | Amount | Calories (kcal) | |
| | | | |
| | | | |
| | | | |
| | | | |
| | | | |
| | Total | | |
| **Lunch** | Amount | Calories (kcal) | |
| | | | |
| | | | |
| | | | |
| | | | |
| | | | |
| | Total | | |

| Snack | Amount | Calories (kcal) |
|---|---|---|
| | | |
| | | |
| | | |
| | Total | |
| Dinner | Amount | Calories (kcal) |
| | | |
| | | |
| | | |
| | | |
| | | |
| | | |
| | | |
| | Total | |
| Snack | Amount | Calories (kcal) |
| | | |
| | | |
| | | |
| | Total | |
| Exercise | Duration | Calories burned (kcal) |
| | | |
| | | |
| | | |
| Water | | Fruit & Veggies | |

Notes:

| Date | S M T W T F S | |
|---|---|---|
| **Breakfast** | Amount | Calories (kcal) |
| | | |
| | | |
| | | |
| | | |
| | | |
| | Total | |
| **Snack** | Amount | Calories (kcal) |
| | | |
| | | |
| | | |
| | | |
| | | |
| | | |
| | Total | |
| **Lunch** | Amount | Calories (kcal) |
| | | |
| | | |
| | | |
| | | |
| | | |
| | Total | |

| Snack | Amount | Calories (kcal) |
|---|---|---|
| | | |
| | | |
| | | |
| | Total | |
| **Dinner** | Amount | Calories (kcal) |
| | | |
| | | |
| | | |
| | | |
| | | |
| | | |
| | | |
| | Total | |
| **Snack** | Amount | Calories (kcal) |
| | | |
| | | |
| | | |
| | Total | |
| **Exercise** | Duration | Calories burned (kcal) |
| | | |
| | | |
| | | |
| **Water** | | Fruit & Veggies | |

Notes:

| Date | S M T W T F S | |
|---|---|---|
| **Breakfast** | Amount | Calories (kcal) |
| | | |
| | | |
| | | |
| | | |
| | | |
| | Total | |
| **Snack** | Amount | Calories (kcal) |
| | | |
| | | |
| | | |
| | | |
| | | |
| | Total | |
| **Lunch** | Amount | Calories (kcal) |
| | | |
| | | |
| | | |
| | | |
| | | |
| | Total | |

| Snack | Amount | Calories (kcal) |
|---|---|---|
| | | |
| | | |
| | | |
| | Total | |
| Dinner | Amount | Calories (kcal) |
| | | |
| | | |
| | | |
| | | |
| | | |
| | | |
| | Total | |
| Snack | Amount | Calories (kcal) |
| | | |
| | | |
| | | |
| | Total | |
| Exercise | Duration | Calories burned (kcal) |
| | | |
| | | |
| | | |

| Water | | | | | | | | Fruit & Veggies | | | | | | | |
|---|---|---|---|---|---|---|---|---|---|---|---|---|---|---|---|

Notes:

| Date | | S M T W T F S |
|---|---|---|
| **Breakfast** | Amount | Calories (kcal) |
| | | |
| | | |
| | | |
| | | |
| | Total | |
| **Snack** | Amount | Calories (kcal) |
| | | |
| | | |
| | | |
| | | |
| | | |
| | | |
| | Total | |
| **Lunch** | Amount | Calories (kcal) |
| | | |
| | | |
| | | |
| | | |
| | | |
| | | |
| | Total | |

| Snack | Amount | Calories (kcal) |
|---|---|---|
|  |  |  |
|  |  |  |
|  |  |  |
|  | Total |  |
| **Dinner** | Amount | Calories (kcal) |
|  |  |  |
|  |  |  |
|  |  |  |
|  |  |  |
|  |  |  |
|  |  |  |
|  |  |  |
|  | Total |  |
| **Snack** | Amount | Calories (kcal) |
|  |  |  |
|  |  |  |
|  |  |  |
|  | Total |  |
| **Exercise** | Duration | Calories burned (kcal) |
|  |  |  |
|  |  |  |
|  |  |  |
| **Water** | | | | | | | | **Fruit & Veggies** | | | | | | | | |

Notes:

| Date | S M T W T F S | |
|---|---|---|
| **Breakfast** | Amount | Calories (kcal) |
| | | |
| | | |
| | | |
| | | |
| | Total | |
| **Snack** | Amount | Calories (kcal) |
| | | |
| | | |
| | | |
| | | |
| | | |
| | Total | |
| **Lunch** | Amount | Calories (kcal) |
| | | |
| | | |
| | | |
| | | |
| | | |
| | Total | |

| Snack | Amount | Calories (kcal) |
|---|---|---|
|  |  |  |
|  |  |  |
|  |  |  |
|  | Total |  |

| Dinner | Amount | Calories (kcal) |
|---|---|---|
|  |  |  |
|  |  |  |
|  |  |  |
|  |  |  |
|  |  |  |
|  |  |  |
|  | Total |  |

| Snack | Amount | Calories (kcal) |
|---|---|---|
|  |  |  |
|  |  |  |
|  |  |  |
|  | Total |  |

| Exercise | Duration | Calories burned (kcal) |
|---|---|---|
|  |  |  |
|  |  |  |
|  |  |  |

| Water |  |  |  |  |  |  |  |  | Fruit & Veggies |  |  |  |  |  |  |  |  |
|---|---|---|---|---|---|---|---|---|---|---|---|---|---|---|---|---|---|

# Notes:

| Date | | S  M  T  W  T  F  S | |
|---|---|---|---|
| **Breakfast** | Amount | Calories (kcal) | |
| | | | |
| | | | |
| | | | |
| | | | |
| | Total | | |
| **Snack** | Amount | Calories (kcal) | |
| | | | |
| | | | |
| | | | |
| | | | |
| | | | |
| | | | |
| | Total | | |
| **Lunch** | Amount | Calories (kcal) | |
| | | | |
| | | | |
| | | | |
| | | | |
| | | | |
| | | | |
| | Total | | |

| Snack | Amount | Calories (kcal) |
|---|---|---|
| | | |
| | | |
| | | |
| | Total | |
| **Dinner** | Amount | Calories (kcal) |
| | | |
| | | |
| | | |
| | | |
| | | |
| | | |
| | | |
| | Total | |
| **Snack** | Amount | Calories (kcal) |
| | | |
| | | |
| | Total | |
| **Exercise** | Duration | Calories burned (kcal) |
| | | |
| | | |
| | | |
| **Water** | | | | | | | | | Fruit & Veggies | | | | | | | | |

Notes:

| Date | | S M T W T F S | |
|---|---|---|---|
| **Breakfast** | Amount | Calories (kcal) | |
| | | | |
| | | | |
| | | | |
| | | | |
| | | | |
| | Total | | |
| **Snack** | Amount | Calories (kcal) | |
| | | | |
| | | | |
| | | | |
| | | | |
| | | | |
| | | | |
| | Total | | |
| **Lunch** | Amount | Calories (kcal) | |
| | | | |
| | | | |
| | | | |
| | | | |
| | | | |
| | | | |
| | Total | | |

| Snack | Amount | Calories (kcal) |
|---|---|---|
| | | |
| | | |
| | | |
| | Total | |
| Dinner | Amount | Calories (kcal) |
| | | |
| | | |
| | | |
| | | |
| | | |
| | | |
| | | |
| | Total | |
| Snack | Amount | Calories (kcal) |
| | | |
| | | |
| | | |
| | Total | |
| Exercise | Duration | Calories burned (kcal) |
| | | |
| | | |
| | | |
| Water | | Fruit & Veggies | |

Notes:

| Date | | S  M  T  W  T  F  S | |
|---|---|---|---|
| **Breakfast** | | Amount | Calories (kcal) |
| | | | |
| | | | |
| | | | |
| | | | |
| | | | |
| | | Total | |
| **Snack** | | Amount | Calories (kcal) |
| | | | |
| | | | |
| | | | |
| | | | |
| | | | |
| | | | |
| | | Total | |
| **Lunch** | | Amount | Calories (kcal) |
| | | | |
| | | | |
| | | | |
| | | | |
| | | | |
| | | | |
| | | Total | |

| Snack | Amount | Calories (kcal) |
|---|---|---|
|  |  |  |
|  |  |  |
|  |  |  |
|  | Total |  |
| **Dinner** | Amount | Calories (kcal) |
|  |  |  |
|  |  |  |
|  |  |  |
|  |  |  |
|  |  |  |
|  | Total |  |
| **Snack** | Amount | Calories (kcal) |
|  |  |  |
|  |  |  |
|  | Total |  |
| **Exercise** | Duration | Calories burned (kcal) |
|  |  |  |
|  |  |  |
|  |  |  |
| **Water** |  | Fruit & Veggies |  |

Notes:

| Date | | S  M  T  W  T  F  S | |
|---|---|---|---|
| **Breakfast** | | Amount | Calories (kcal) |
| | | | |
| | | | |
| | | | |
| | | | |
| | | Total | |
| **Snack** | | Amount | Calories (kcal) |
| | | | |
| | | | |
| | | | |
| | | | |
| | | | |
| | | Total | |
| **Lunch** | | Amount | Calories (kcal) |
| | | | |
| | | | |
| | | | |
| | | | |
| | | | |
| | | Total | |

| Snack | Amount | Calories (kcal) |
|---|---|---|
|  |  |  |
|  |  |  |
|  |  |  |
|  | Total |  |
| **Dinner** | Amount | Calories (kcal) |
|  |  |  |
|  |  |  |
|  |  |  |
|  |  |  |
|  |  |  |
|  |  |  |
|  |  |  |
|  | Total |  |
| **Snack** | Amount | Calories (kcal) |
|  |  |  |
|  |  |  |
|  |  |  |
|  | Total |  |
| **Exercise** | Duration | Calories burned (kcal) |
|  |  |  |
|  |  |  |
|  |  |  |
| **Water** |  | Fruit & Veggies |

# Notes:

| Date | | S  M  T  W  T  F  S | |
|---|---|---|---|
| **Breakfast** | | Amount | Calories (kcal) |
| | | | |
| | | | |
| | | | |
| | | | |
| | | | |
| | | Total | |
| **Snack** | | Amount | Calories (kcal) |
| | | | |
| | | | |
| | | | |
| | | | |
| | | | |
| | | | |
| | | Total | |
| **Lunch** | | Amount | Calories (kcal) |
| | | | |
| | | | |
| | | | |
| | | | |
| | | | |
| | | | |
| | | Total | |

| Snack | Amount | Calories (kcal) |
|---|---|---|
| | | |
| | | |
| | | |
| | Total | |
| **Dinner** | Amount | Calories (kcal) |
| | | |
| | | |
| | | |
| | | |
| | | |
| | | |
| | | |
| | Total | |
| **Snack** | Amount | Calories (kcal) |
| | | |
| | | |
| | | |
| | Total | |
| **Exercise** | Duration | Calories burned (kcal) |
| | | |
| | | |
| | | |

| Water | | | | | | | | | Fruit & Veggies | | | | | | | | |
|---|---|---|---|---|---|---|---|---|---|---|---|---|---|---|---|---|---|

www.ingramcontent.com/pod-product-compliance
Lightning Source LLC
Chambersburg PA
CBHW051352280526
45784CB00007B/2920